1

INTRODUCTION

A prominent player in the complex world of antimicrobial drugs, ciprofloxacin is an antibiotic belonging to the fluoroquinolone class, which is renowned for its ability to kill a wide variety of bacteria. Ciprofloxacin was born out of a desperate need for antibiotics that could kill a broad variety of bacteria. Its invention and subsequent discovery were watershed moments in the study of infectious diseases, strengthening the toolbox for combating bacterial enemies.

The Core of Ciprofloxacin: The synthetic fluoroquinolone ciprofloxacin exerts its antibacterial power by means of a process intricately connected to the genetic machinery of bacteria. Ciprofloxacin slows or stops the development of bacteria by blocking two enzymes that are crucial for DNA replication and repair: bacterial DNA gyrase and topoisomerase IV. Its versatility as a clinician's toolkit is highlighted by its unusual mechanism, which makes it effective against both Gram-negative and certain Gram-positive bacteria.

The therapeutic landscape in which ciprofloxacin acts is complex and wide-ranging. Infections of the respiratory, urinary, cutaneous, soft tissue, gastrointestinal, and skeletal systems are all possible signs. Ciprofloxacin is a wonderful ally in the fight against all kinds of bacteria, whether you're dealing with difficult UTIs or community-acquired pneumonia.

The intricacies of ciprofloxacin's dosage and administration must be fully grasped in order to navigate the dosing seas. It goes beyond milligrams when it comes to dosing considerations; it is available in both oral and intravenous versions. The intricate story of therapeutic precision is woven by dose modifications according to the severity of the illness, considerations for pediatric and geriatric groups, and the significance of adherence. By navigating these dosage waters, healthcare providers aim for the best possible patient outcomes while minimizing the chances of resistance and side effects.

While we strive for therapeutic success, the prospect of undesirable reactions looms large. The careful balance between benefit and risk could be disrupted as ciprofloxacin's adverse effects unfold across the body, from the intestines to the brain. Antibiotic stewards must be ever-vigilant in the face of infrequent but severe adverse events, photosensitivity, tendon ruptures, and other similar issues.

Antimicrobial Resistance and Ciprofloxacin: As we explore ciprofloxacin, we face the dynamic story of antibiotic resistance. Ciprofloxacin, which was once a strong protector, is now under attack from bacteria that are resistant to it. This has us thinking about ways to keep it effective. Responsible antibiotic usage becomes a narrative that relies heavily on surveillance, careful prescribing, and ongoing research.

Beyond the present therapeutic landscape, the unwritten future of ciprofloxacin is full of questions and opportunities. New aspects of its pharmacology are being investigated through ongoing research and clinical studies, which may lead to advancements in fluoroquinolone treatment. The next chapter in the story of ciprofloxacin will be filled out as we approach the dawn of a new day.

We will explore the pharmacological pathways, therapeutic settings, and significant influence of ciprofloxacin in protecting human health from bacterial threats.

POSSIBLE SIGNIFICANCE

When it comes to treating bacterial infections, the versatile broad-spectrum fluoroquinolone antibiotic ciprofloxacin really shines. Its versatility and effectiveness against a vast array of bacterial infections are reflected in its indications, which span many organ systems.

1. When it comes to fighting off diseases of the respiratory system, ciprofloxacin is an absolute lifesaver. This includes illnesses of the lower and upper respiratory tracts. Its effectiveness covers a

range of Gram-negative and certain Gram-positive bacteria that are frequently associated with diseases like chronic bronchitis and community-acquired pneumonia.

2. With its remarkable effectiveness against uropathogenic bacteria, ciprofloxacin has become an essential component in the treatment of urinary tract infections (UTIs). It works wonders on both severe and mild UTIs thanks to its capacity to

reach high concentrations in the urinary system.

3. diseases of the GI Tract: Ciprofloxacin treats bacterial gastroenteritis caused by Shigella and Salmonella among other GI tract diseases. It is a great alternative for moderate to severe bacterial gastroenteritis because it can be taken orally and treated without the need for hospitalization.

4. Ciprofloxacin is effective against a wide variety of skin and soft

tissue infections, including those caused by some Gram-negative bacteria and Staphylococcus aureus strains that are susceptible to it. This tool is useful for a wide range of diseases, including simple skin infections, cellulitis, and wound infections.

5. Infections of the Bones and Joints: Ciprofloxacin is used to treat some types of infections of the musculoskeletal system. It is efficient against bacterial infections that cause osteomyelitis and septic arthritis because it penetrates bone tissues.

6. Ciprofloxacin is not only used to treat the aforementioned illnesses, but also for a wide range of additional infections, such as those involving the abdomen or the genitourinary system, where its spectrum of action coincides with that of the infectious agents responsible.

With its wide range of uses, ciprofloxacin is an important part of the treatment arsenal, giving doctors a weapon against bacterial infections in various parts of the body. To optimize therapeutic outcomes and reduce the evolution of antibiotic resistance, it is vital to use antibiotics prudently, guided by microbial susceptibility tests and assessments of local resistance patterns.

ADMINISTRATION & DOSAGE

To get the most out of ciprofloxacin—a fluoroquinolone antibiotic known for its broad-spectrum activity—and to avoid side effects and antibiotic resistance, dosing and administration must be carefully considered.

1. Dosage and Administration Methods:

Tablets and oral solution are two examples of the oral forms of ciprofloxacin that allow for treatment of a variety of infections to be done outside of a hospital setting.

When oral administration is not an option due to a severe infection or other medical reason, intravenous ciprofloxacin formulations provide a more reliable and faster drug delivery system.

2. Considerations for Dosage:

The dosage of ciprofloxacin is usually determined by the kind and severity of the infection. A smaller dose may be enough for mild to moderate infections, but higher doses may be necessary for severe infections.

Particular Infections: It is vital to adjust the dosage according to the particular infection. Dosage recommendations for respiratory infections and UTIs, for example, could be different.

3. Issues Relevant to Children:

Pediatric dosing necessitates meticulous deliberation, with modifications being implemented in accordance with the child's age, weight, and the particular infection that is being addressed. Oral suspensions and other pediatric formulations are available to help with precise dosage in this group.

4. Issues related to the elderly:

Dosage adjustments may be required in the elderly due to possible changes in renal function related with aging. It is essential to closely monitor renal function in order to prevent the medication from building up.

5. Following the Recommended Protocol:

Even if symptoms improve before the recommended course of ciprofloxacin is finished, patients are still urged to finish the entire course. This guarantees total infection elimination and aids in preventing drug resistance.

6. Things to Keep in Mind Regarding Drug Interactions:

When taken with other medications, ciprofloxacin's absorption can be affected. This is especially true when the other prescription contains divalent or trivalent cations, such as magnesium, calcium, or aluminum. Maintaining therapeutic efficacy requires understanding potential medication interactions.

7. Reasons Why Prompt Administration Is Crucial:

Maintaining a regular interval between doses is vital for oral formulations to achieve therapeutic medication levels. regular timing is also important. To prevent side effects, it is important to administer intravenous medications at the prescribed infusion rates.

8. Keep an eye on:

Renal Function: People at risk of renal impairment or who already have renal problems should have their renal function monitored regularly.

When it comes to keeping drug concentrations within the target therapeutic range, therapeutic drug monitoring can be a lifesaver.

Accurate therapeutic dosing and administration of ciprofloxacin relies heavily on the expertise of healthcare providers. To achieve the best possible patient outcomes when using this fluoroquinolone, it is necessary to adapt the regimen based on the infection's specifics, patient considerations, and close monitoring.

POTENTIAL SIDE EFFECTS

The possible negative effects of ciprofloxacin, a fluoroquinolone antibiotic highly regarded for its broad-spectrum activity, must be carefully considered. A careful balancing act between therapeutic effectiveness and the prudent control of adverse effects must be achieved as clinicians utilize its potency to fight bacterial infections.

1. Health Impact on the Digestive System:

Typical side effects include feeling sick to your stomach, throwing up, and nausea. In many cases, these effects can be alleviated by taking ciprofloxacin with food.

2. Neurological System Impacts:

Insomnia, vertigo, and headaches are common side effects. Patients should be careful not to do anything that could put their mental alertness at risk.

3. Tendonitis and Rupture:

Ciprofloxacin causes an increased chance of tendon ruptures, especially in the Achilles tendon, which is rare but serious. Patients using corticosteroids at the same time or who are elderly are at a higher risk.

4. Exposure to light

Sunburn is more likely to occur in patients who have an increased sensitivity to sunlight. It is advised to use sunscreen and protective gear to adequately shield oneself from the sun.

5. Responses to Allergens:

Allergic reactions, which are extremely rare but can cause serious symptoms like swelling, itching, and skin rash, are possible. Though they are uncommon, severe allergic responses can cause anaphylaxis, which necessitates rapid medical intervention.

6. Systemic and Gastrointestinal Infections:

Possible Side Effects: Bacterial or fungal infections that are resistant to ciprofloxacin can develop in the digestive tract and other organs if the drug is administered for an extended period of time. Treatment and post-treatment monitoring for secondary infections is of the utmost importance.

7. Diarrhea caused by Clostridium difficile:

Ciprofloxacin seldom causes serious side effects, including Clostridium difficile-associated diarrhea (CD), which can be mild or even fatal. Constant bowel movement monitoring and prompt treatment are of the utmost importance.

8. Damage to the liver:

Hepatotoxicity and elevated liver enzymes are extremely rare but potentially fatal side effects. It is especially important to keep an eye on individuals who already have liver problems when they are on ciprofloxacin.

9. Medication Interactions:

Potential Drug Interactions: Ciprofloxacin has the ability to change the way other drugs work or perhaps make them less safe to use. It is critical to pay close attention to drug interactions, particularly with drugs that impact the central nervous system.

10. Effects on the Musculoskeletal System in Children:

Cause for Concern in Pediatrics: There may be musculoskeletal side effects from using ciprofloxacin in children. The use of this medication in children is often restricted for special cases and is subject to thorough evaluation.

Accurate knowledge of possible side effects is critical for doctors navigating the ciprofloxacin therapeutic landscape. To administer this potent antibiotic responsibly and effectively, it is necessary to tailor treatment to specific patient profiles, monitor for early symptoms of adverse effects, and carefully assess the risks and benefits. An important part of establishing a cooperative strategy for antimicrobial treatment is educating patients about the risks of the medication and the need of reporting any unexpected symptoms immediately.

SUBSTANCE INTERACTIONS

Understanding Ciprofloxacin Interactions: A Detour Through Pharmacological Networks

Healthcare practitioners must exercise caution while prescribing the powerful fluoroquinolone antibiotic ciprofloxacin due to the drug's intricate network of interactions. Understanding these interactions is crucial for doctors navigating the pharmaceutical landscape, as it allows them to optimize treatment outcomes while minimizing the risk of side effects and impaired efficacy.

1. Multivalent Cation Interactions:

Coadministration of ciprofloxacin with antacids, calcium, magnesium, or aluminum-containing medications may reduce the drug's absorption. Take ciprofloxacin at least 2 hours prior to or 6 hours following the administration of these products to reduce the likelihood of an interaction.

2. Sucralfate Interaction:

Concurrent usage of sucralfate may decrease the absorption of ciprofloxacin. To prevent this interaction, give them at least two hours apart.

3. Iron Supplement Interactions:

Ciprofloxacin absorption may be impaired if you use iron supplements. To get the best results, give these agents at least a few hours apart.

4. Related to Warfarin:

Because of its anticoagulant properties, ciprofloxacin raises the risk of bleeding when taken with warfarin. Time to thrombin and international normalized ratio (INR) must be closely monitored.

5. How Theophylline Interacts:

Sera Theophylline Levels: Ciprofloxacin has the ability to raise theophylline levels, which may result in harmful effects. It is advised to adjust the dosage of the theophylline and keep an eye on serum levels.

6. The following medications interact with NSAIDs:

Using ciprofloxacin with nonsteroidal anti-inflammatory drugs (NSAIDs) at the same time may increase the likelihood of seizures. People who have had seizures in the past should use extra caution.

7. How Anti-Diabetic Medication Interacts:

The risk of hypoglycemia increases when taking ciprofloxacin since it may increase the efficacy of antidiabetic drugs. It may be required to monitor blood glucose levels and make adjustments to the dosages of antidiabetic medication.

8. How Methotrexate Interacts:

Ciprofloxacin raises the risk of methotrexate poisoning by increasing methotrexate levels. Dosage adjustments and side effect monitoring with methotrexate should be prioritized.

9. Drug Interactions with CNS Substances:

The central nervous system (CNS) effects of ciprofloxacin may be amplified when used with other drugs that have an effect on the CNS, such as antidepressants or antipsychotics. People who are already at a higher risk should use extra caution.

10. Corticosteroids and Their Interactions:

The risk of tendon rupture may be increased when ciprofloxacin and corticosteroids are used together, particularly in older patients. You need to be careful when using this combination.

To ensure the safe and effective administration of ciprofloxacin, it is crucial to understand these medication interactions. To reduce the likelihood of adverse drug reactions, healthcare practitioners should do comprehensive medication evaluations, take specific patient characteristics into account, and communicate clearly with patients. Comprehensive and patient-centered treatment is enhanced by routine changes to a patient's pharmaceutical profile, which includes over-the-counter and herbal medications.

THE END

final thought

Conclusion: Ciprofloxacin's Role in the Therapeutic Odyssey

In the complex realm of antibiotic treatment, the story of ciprofloxacin is both an exciting adventure and a calculated risk-taking maneuver against infectious illnesses. Now that we have covered all there is to know about this fluoroquinolone, it is important to think about its many functions, both positive and negative, in the context of antimicrobial stewardship.

Advantages of Ciprofloxacin:

Ciprofloxacin is an invaluable ally in the fight against germs due to its broad-spectrum activity and adaptable formulations. Its effectiveness extends across a wide variety of therapeutic contexts, including infections of the respiratory system, urinary tract, skin, and soft tissues. Its versatility is enhanced by the fact that it may be easily administered orally or intravenously, making it suitable for use in outpatient settings for infections that are not too serious and offering a strong intravenous alternative for those that are.

Things to Think About and Overcome:

Ciprofloxacin resistance is a real possibility during treatment. Careful evaluation is required in light of the potential for adverse reactions, which can range from mild nausea and vomiting to more severe and uncommon consequences such tendon ruptures and hepatotoxicity. Healthcare providers are always faced with the dilemma of how to treat present infections while also ensuring that antibiotics like ciprofloxacin remain effective for generations to come, all because of the advent of antibiotic resistance.

How to Use Antibiotics Responsibly:

Understanding ciprofloxacin's intricacies puts the practice of prudent antibiotic use front and center. When it comes to finding the sweet spot between therapeutic efficacy and risk minimization, healthcare providers are indispensable. Important parts of this duty include adapting the dosage to the particular infection, taking patient characteristics into account, and carefully watching for side effects. An integral part of the therapy process is educating patients on the significance of reporting any unexpected symptoms quickly and finishing the entire treatment regimen.

Drug Interactions: A Comprehensive Guide

The complex network of medication interactions highlights the importance of cautious navigation even more. Clinicians must exercise extreme caution when prescribing ciprofloxacin because of the drug's interaction with other drugs, including anticoagulants and multivalent cations. To ensure a safe and effective treatment journey, it is essential to assess medications often, communicate with patients about their full pharmaceutical profile, and be mindful of possible interactions.

In the Future:

As we wrap off this chapter on ciprofloxacin, it's important to look ahead to what's to come. The pharmacology of fluoroquinolones is still a mystery, but ongoing studies and clinical trials should shed light on some of those mysteries. As new obstacles arise in the course of antimicrobial treatment, healthcare practitioners are urged to keep their wits about them, be flexible, and stay educated.

In this final section, we acknowledge the importance of ciprofloxacin and its impact on infectious disorders, but we also acknowledge that we must all exercise caution while using this powerful medication. An essential part of the story of antibiotic use, the journey with ciprofloxacin exemplifies the never-ending drive for better treatments and the never-ending fight against infectious diseases.

At the Extreme

Made in the USA
Las Vegas, NV
08 March 2024

86907707R00036